YOUR KNOWLEDGE HAS VALUE

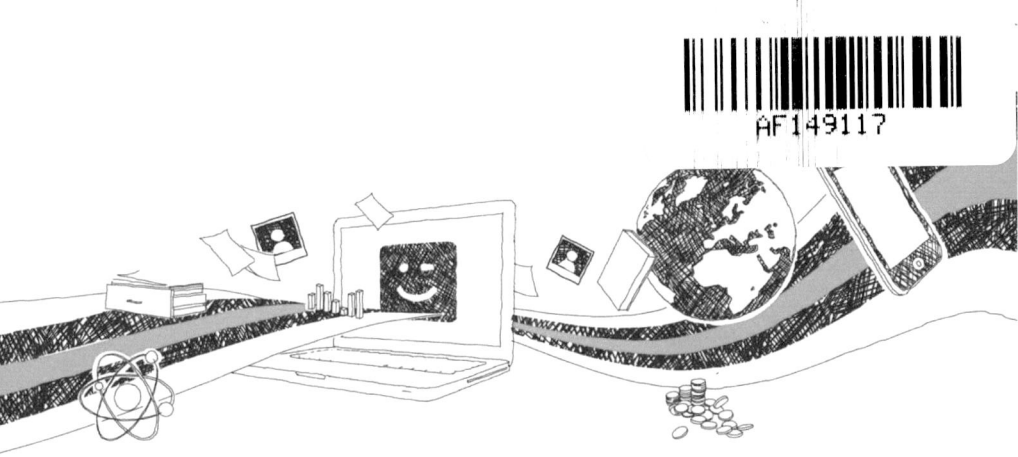

- We will publish your bachelor's and master's thesis, essays and papers

- Your own eBook and book - sold worldwide in all relevant shops

- Earn money with each sale

Upload your text at www.GRIN.com
and publish for free

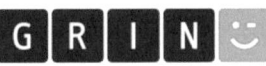

Klaus Schöfer

Clinical Risk Management: What measures are available to hospital managers in order to control the frequency of clinical negligence claims and their ultimate cost? To what extent can they transfer that risk to others?

Examicus Verlag

Bibliographic information published by the German National Library:

The German National Library lists this publication in the National Bibliography; detailed bibliographic data are available on the Internet at http://dnb.dnb.de .

Copyright © 1998 GRIN Verlag GmbH
Print and binding: Books on Demand GmbH, Norderstedt Germany
ISBN: 978-3-656-99140-3

Examicus - Verlag für akademische Texte

Der Examicus Verlag mit Sitz in München hat sich auf die Veröffentlichung akademischer Texte spezialisiert.

Die Verlagswebseite www.examicus.de ist für Studenten, Hochschullehrer und andere Akademiker die ideale Plattform, ihre Fachtexte, Studienarbeiten, Abschlussarbeiten oder Dissertationen einem breiten Publikum zu präsentieren.

"What measures are available to hospital managers in order to control the frequency of clinical negligence claims and their ultimate cost? To what extent can they transfer that risk to others? Illustrate your answers with examples from either the UK or US health care sectors."

Name: Klaus Schoefer

Department: School of Management and Finance

Module Title: Risk Management

Coursework to be submitted: Essay

Contents

1. Introduction

The purpose of the present paper is to examine measures, available to hospital managers to control the frequency of clinical negligence claims and their ultimate cost. Moreover, the extent to which hospital managers can transfer that risk to others is investigated. As such, the paper is divided into three parts. First, the need for clinical risk management is established. This is followed by a brief account of the main aspects within clinical risk management: Financial Control, Claim Management and Claim Prevention. Finally, an outline of the insurance-prevention trade-off and its impact on the transference of risk is provided.

2. The Need for Clinical Risk Management

The last two decades have witnessed a sharp increase in the frequency and severity of medical negligence claims. As a matter of fact, medical practitioners had to face a serious rise in the cost of their malpractice insurance (Danzon, 1985; Dingwall and Fenn, 1991). In the UK, for example, subscription rates paid to one of the three defence organisations, rose from ≤ 264 in 1984 to ≤ 1080 in 1988 (Dingwall and Fenn, 1991). Under the condition of NHS employment, it was not possible to pass these cost increases on to patients and these costs were directly born by physicians. The problem got even bigger when defence organisations introduced a speciality-rated premium structure. Within this framework, considerable variations in residual income by speciality had to be feared, since hospital doctors are paid on a common scale. The Department of Health, finally, decided to resolve this matter by abrogating its agreement that tort liability is to be shared with doctors. From April 1991, clinical negligence liability was transferred to Trusts and Directly Managed Units, as the actual employers of medical staff (Fenn and Hodges, 1997; Dingwall and Fenn, 1991). These cost pressures, actual and potential, on health authority budgets were a sufficient incentive for British providers to concern themselves with the potential of risk management to control their losses from negligence litigation. In this context, the financial impact of large settlements is of particular importance (Fenn and Dingwall, 1991). Although it can be softened by loan arrangements, there is still concern over their potential disruption to the planning of patient care (Fenn and Hodges, 1997).

Apart from financial costs, there are other reasons why a hospital manager should be concerned about risk management. 'Adverse events' also involve huge personal cost to the people involved. Often, patients suffer from increased pain, disability, and psychological trauma and may experience their treatment as a betrayal of trust. They may become angry, depressed, and bitter, and their problems are often compounded by a protracted adversarial legal process (Vincent, 1995a; Vincent, 1995b). Staff, on the other hand, may experience guilt, shame, and depression after making a mistake. Litigation and complaints impose an additional burden on them. A doctor, for example, whose confidence has been reduced will probably work less effectively and efficiently. Sometimes, doctors even abandon medicine as a career (Vincent, 1995b; Genn, 1995).

3. Clinical Risk Management

Risk Management can be broadly defined as the reduction of harm to an organisation, by identifying and, as far as possible eliminating risk. In a clinical setting, the primary focus is on malpractice, which causes financial losses but also affects the reputation and morale of a trust and its staff. Clinical risk management also involves the continuing care of the injured patients and rapid settlement of justified claims (Clements, 1995). According to a working definition by Dingwall and Fenn (1991), the aim of clinical risk management is threefold:

(1) Prediction of losses and ensuring that adequate levels of reserves have been allocated to meet them.
(2) Active management in order either to prevent the lodging of a claim or to promote an early resolution which will limit the legal costs.
(3) Review of data on claims made as evidence of points of weakness in service or clinical practice which can be remedied by executive or professional action.

3.1 Financial Control

Following a traditional insurance industry sense, hospital managers seek to project the likely costs of negligence claims against their institution in order to make accurate cash provision from one year to another (Dingwall and Fenn, 1991). However, due to shifts in the success rate of claimants and the unpredictable incidence of high-value cases, this exercise seems unlikely to justify much expenditure. If liability is fixed on units, as regulated in the 1991 version of NHS Indemnity, unit treasurers may see their liability fluctuate widely from a few thousand to several million and back again from one year to the next (Dingwall and Fenn, 1991; Fenn and Hodges, 1997). Although this could be balanced to some extend by a loan scheme, allowing units to borrow money from Regions, the numbers are too small to smooth out these random elements. Consequently, a compilation of claims at this level yields too few cases to sustain any kind of sophisticated risk analysis. From an insurance perspective, Regional pools are unsatisfactory, District pools are unrealistic and unit liability is absurd. In Dingwall and Fenn's (1991) view, the compilation of a computerised database can only be done at a national level and people would be better employed trying to make that happen.

3.2 Claim Management

As mentioned before, another dimension of clinical risk management is the active management of claims to reduce the chance of litigation or to reduce the costs. In this context, it is important to focus on the way in which a hospital manager responses to litigation. When a 'letter before action' is received, the hospital manager should determine the response of the trust. As Clements (1995) points out, it is important to remember that often the injured patient seeks only an explanation and an apology and is not primarily motivated by money. In many cases the matter is trivial, issues are clear cut, and an offer of a very modest settlement may deflect a potentially costly legal action. This is consistent with US data, according to which more than 90 per cent of claims are settled out of court. Of these, about half are dropped without payment. The other half were settled for an average of $ 26,000, far less than the $ 102,000 average award in the small minority of tried cases that the plaintiff won (Danzon, 1985).

Litigation has shortcomings both for patients and practitioners. As Brown and Simanowitz (1995) point out, the public perception for patients is that the most serious failings are cost and delay. Due to the reduction in the availability of legal aid very few ordinary families can afford to undertake medical negligence litigation. Even the move towards conditional fees ("no win, no fee") is only superficially attractive since the plaintiff remains at risk of paying the huge costs of the defendants in the event of the action failing. Furthermore, solicitors are likely to undertake only cases with high success probabilities. Delay, unlike cost, may not actually deny justice to patients but causes immense distress and hardship. Brown and Simanowitz (1995) report that the average time before a medical negligence case in the UK is resolved is about four years. During this time, the patient and his/her dependants may suffer considerable privation. Similarly, doctors interviewed who had experienced being the subject of a medical negligence action found the experience to some extent distressing at the time (Genn, 1995; Brown and Simanowitz, 1995; Ennis and Grudzinskas, 1993).

Accordingly, in common with other fields of activity, there have been moves to seek alternatives to litigation for medical disputes by using processes which effectively serve many of the functions of litigation but with the opportunity to avoid some of its negative consequences. These processes make use of a neutral who impartially helps the parties to resolve their dispute. Two fundamentally different ways have to be distinguished: First adjudication, in which the neutral makes a decision which is binding on both sides, and second, non-adjudicatory alternative dispute resolution, in which the neutral has no authority to make any binding decision but instead helps the parties to arrive at their own binding agreement (Brown and Simanowitz, 1995). The most popular adjudicatory forms of alternative dispute resolution in the medical context are arbitration and expert determination. Non-adjudicatory, or consensual, forms include pre-trial screening panels, mediation and the mini-trial. For the purpose of this paper, however, I shall expand only on arbitration and pre-trial screening panels.

Adjudication of Medical Disputes: Arbitration

Arbitration is a well-used voluntary procedure whereby patients and health care providers may enter into written agreements for the submission of any disputes or claims to a third party. The third party is neutral, selected by the parties or through some agreed selection procedure, hears and determines the issues, and makes a binding decision. The quality of the arbitrator's approach can be judicial, but the procedures and rules of evidence may be simplified from the traditional court process, and special rules may be applied (Warren, 1980; Danzon, 1985; Brown and Simanowitz, 1995) In some cases, for example, the arbitrator may be assisted by an expert medical assessor. In the UK arbitration services are available for medical claim. For instance, the Chartered Institute of Arbitrators has developed an arbitration scheme for medical negligence claims within the NHS (Brown and Simanowitz, 1995). However, there are also concerns about arbitration, especially in the case where a medical provider has sufficient monopoly power to force arbitration on patients as a precondition of providing services, or if patients are uninformed. Suppliers of arbitration services would then have incentives to design procedures in favour of doctors. Consequently, many patients' groups do not consider arbitration being an attractive proposition (Brown and Simanowitz, 1995; Danzon, 1985). This is consistent with US NAIC data on claims in the period 1975-1978, which reports that only one-third of one per cent were closed by arbitration. However, the data also shows a higher plaintiff win rate and lower award in arbitration than in court (Danzon, 1985).

Another mechanism designed as an alternative to trial, is the pre-trial screening panel. In the US, these panels are typically composed of three to seven members, including a solicitor, a doctor (usually of the same speciality as the defendant) and a judge or solicitor chairman appointed by the court. Normally, the hearing conducted by the panel is informal, and the strict rules of evidence on the claim are not applicable. The panel's decision is not binding on the parties, and it does not preclude any party from initiating a lawsuit. However, to discourage further litigation, some statutes may impose penalties against a party who rejects the panel finding and fails to prevail at trial (Warren, 1980; Danzon, 1985)

Proponents of panels hoped that an early review of cases by an informal panel of experts would facilitate fair and speedy disposition of claims. Theory and evidence, on the other hand, suggest that the panel model may have severe drawbacks. Rational litigants are supposed to continue to trial if the cost of proceeding are less than the difference between the expectations of the outcome. A panel, however, will narrow divergence of expectations about the outcome at verdict only if it is a reasonable replication of a jury trial. This implies using formal rule of evidence and allowing full discovery which entails the costs and delay that the panel are intended to prevent. Moreover, once the costs of a panel hearing have been incurred, the incremental costs of proceeding to trial are reduced, which in turn tends to encourage litigation. Finally, pre-trial panels may reduce the plaintiff's chances in subsequent appeals as US data proves (Danzon, 1985).

3.3 Claim Prevention

The third aspect of clinical risk management, claim prevention, asks whether claims data can contribute to quality improvement. More specifically, does the claims data contain any information that could be used in order to identify potential claimants or risky areas and help to defuse them? The Oxford Region study, for example, found that only five specialities account for almost two-thirds of all claims made and paid. This seems to be a sufficiently limited target to encourage an investigation of risky events (Dingwall and Fenn, 1991). However, it is important to have a realistic view of what is achievable. Dingwall and Fenn (1991), for example, stress that there is evidence to suggest that the rise in medical negligence litigation in the UK may have more to do with external factors to the health care system than to changes in behaviour of the system or its personal which could be influenced by internal measures.

Having said that, I shall now focus on what can be done at a local level? Three types of activities seem to be practicable and worth exploring:

First, the creation of a 'culture of safety' in health care. This approach has become increasingly influential due to the evident limitations of purely rule-based or technological solutions to risk problems. It is important to make the staff sensitive to the early identification of trouble and to encourage a more reflective response. It may, for example, involve managers and doctors being more explicit with each other and with patients about the balance of risk inherent in health care (Dingwall and Fenn, 1991). The 'culture of safety' should also involve the attempt to make positive use of the information which claims represent about the quality of care. Consequently, each claim should be treated as the basis of a comprehensive inquiry into the possible sources for poor organisational and individual performance. Investigations, in this context, can be seen as a mode of quality improvement rather than a device to allocate blame (Dingwall and Fenn, 1991). Finally, proactive claim management has to be mentioned. The philosophy of this concept is that medical care providers should observe and immediately report deviations from expected outcomes and any hospital acquired patient injury with liability potential. This in turn triggers immediate investigation in cases with liability potential and active intervention to assist the patient. In California institutions in which this proactive approach has been operational, a risk management team can be alerted to any mishap and immediately become responsible for freezing key documentation, taking statements and supervising patient relations (Lindgren and Secker-Walker, 1995; Dingwall and Fenn, 1991). Medical mishaps become an occasion for the hospital to demonstrate goodwill by a speedy admission of fault where justified and to work with the patients to identify economic losses and to make an early and realistic offer of settlement (Dingwall and Fenn, 1991). "Whether or not such a policy .. weakens the bargaining position of the Trusts ... is something which needs to be examined further." (Fenn and Hodges, 1997, p. 241)

4. The Transference of Risk

One of the most important clinical risk management decisions made by hospital managers is the extent to which risk is transferred to another party such as a insurance company. In order to answer this question I shall first address the role of liability insurance and its effect on prevention in the context of medical malpractice.

The problem of a malpractice claim depends partly on unpredictable effects of treatment and on whims of patients and courts, but also on the care of the physician. Liability insurance for doctors may therefore be undesirable since it reduces incentives for prevention (Danzon, 1985). On the other hand, liability insurance is needed since it protects doctors. Having said that, it becomes clear that determining the optimal level of insurance coverage (or risk retention respectively) is an issue. In this context, perfect experience rating is often advocated as a solution to the moral hazard problem (Danzon, 1985; Sloan, 1990). Insurance would still provide protection when a loss occurs, but incentives to invest optimally in loss reduction are preserved. Perfect experience rating, however, is infeasible because insurers lack the information to distinguish valid from invalid claims. Therefore, in practice, most lines of insurance adopt a second-best solution: the insured retains some financial stake in the loss through a deductible, a coinsurance percentage, or a premium that is merit-rated on the basis of claim experience. Incentives for loss prevention, albeit reduced, can so be preserved by financial exposure. Evidence on malpractice insurance contracts, however, shows that such forms of risk retention appear to be relatively uncommon; the typical malpractice insurance policy provides virtually complete coverage of monetary losses (Danzon, 1985).

Once the institutional decision about where losses should fall has been determined, it is then up to the parties concerned whether or not to make arrangements to spread, or pool, the losses through insurance (Fenn, 1993). If risk averse, patients may purchase first-party insurance against the losses they have to bear themselves. Doctors, on the other hand, may purchase third-party liability insurance against the cost of meeting patient claims. As an alternative, they could form mutual societies for the pooling of such losses (Danzon, 1985; Fenn, 1993). In the US, for example, doctors play an active role on the supply side of the market both in the programmes sponsored by the medical society and written by stock carriers and in the case of physician-owned companies (Danzon, 1985). In the UK, the Clinical Negligence Scheme for Trusts (CNST), which is operating since April 1995, is a means by which a Trust can share the risk of large claims with other Trusts through contribution to a mutual fund (Fenn and Hodges, 1997)

5. Conclusion

To sum up, the sharp increase in both the frequency and severity of medical malpractice claims has fostered the need for clinical risk management. The aims of clinical risk management are (1) to reduce the frequency of adverse events, (2) to reduce the chance of a claim being made, and (3) to control the cost of claims that are made. Finally, the extent to which clinical risk is transferred to others, has to be seen within a insurance-prevention trade-off-context.

References

Brown, H. and Simanowitz, A. (1995) 'Alternative dispute resolution and mediation', in C. Vincent (ed.), *Clinical Risk Management*, London: BMJ Publications.

Clements, R. V. (1995) 'Essentials of clinical risk management', in C. Vincent (ed.), *Clinical Risk Management*, London: BMJ Publications.

Danzon, P. M. (1985) *Medical Malpractice: Theory, Evidence, and Public Policy*, Cambridge, Massachusetts: Harvard University Press.

Dingwall, R. and Fenn, P. (1991) 'Is risk management necessary?', *International Journal of Risk & Safety in Medicine*, 2, 91-106.

Ennis, M. and Grudzinskas, J. G. (1993) 'The effect of accidents and litigation on doctors', in C. Vincent, M. Ennis and R. J. Audley (eds.), *Medical Accidents*, Oxford: Oxford University Press.

Fenn, P. (1993) 'Compensation for medical injury: a review of policy options', in C. Vincent, M. Ennis and R. J. Audley (eds.), *Medical Accidents*, Oxford: Oxford University Press.

Fenn, P. and Hodges, R. (1997) 'Long-tail Liabilities and Claims Management in the NHS', in R. Baldwin (ed.), *Law and Uncertainty*, Kluwer Academic Press.

Genn, H. (1995) 'Supporting staff involved in litigation', in C. Vincent (ed.), *Clinical Risk Management*, London: BMJ Publications.

Lindgren, O. and Secker-Walker, J. (1995) 'Incident reporting systems: early warnings for the prevention and control of clinical negligence', in C. Vincent (ed.), *Clinical Risk Management*, London: BMJ Publications.

Sloan, F. A. (1990) 'Experience Rating: Does it Make Sense for Medical Malpractice Insurance?', *American Economic Review*, 80(2), 128-133.

Vincent, C. (1995a) 'Introduction', in C. Vincent (ed.), *Clinical Risk Management*, London: BMJ Publications.

Vincent, C. (1995b) 'Caring for patients harmed by treatment', in C. Vincent (ed.), *Clinical Risk Management*, London: BMJ Publications.

Warren, D. G. (1980) 'Medical Malpractice in the United States of America', in J. L. Taylor (ed.), *Medical Malpractice*, Bristol: John Wright & Sons Ltd.